I0697449

Overcoming Hemorrhagic Stroke
(Intracerebral Hemorrhage)

A Complete Patient's Guide to Treat Hemorrhagic Stroke, Causes, Preventive Measures, Emergency Treatment and Management

Dan Phillips PhD

~DEDICATION~

~LARRY~

For your unwavering support, encouragement, and friendship. Your presence in my life has been a constant source of inspiration. Thank you for your invaluable kindness and belief in my journey. This book is a token of appreciation for your enduring friendship and steadfast encouragement.

TABLE OF CONTENT

DEDICATION   **1**

TABLE OF CONTENT   **2**

°°PART I: UNDERSTANDING HEMORRHAGIC STROKE°°

1. UNDERSTANDING HEMORRHAGIC STROKE: AN OVERVIEW
   ° DEFINITION OF HEMORRHAGIC STROKE
   ° TYPES OF HEMORRHAGIC STROKE
   ° PREVALENCE OF HEMORRHAGIC STROKE

°°PART II: CAUSES AND RISK FACTORS°°

2. UNRAVELING THE CAUSES: WHAT TRIGGERS HEMORRHAGIC STROKE?
   ° HYPERTENSION
   ° ANEURYSMS
   ° BLOOD THINNERS
   ° GENETIC PREDISPOSITIONS
   ° OTHER RISK FACTORS

°°Part III: Signs and Symptoms°°

3. Signs and Symptoms: Recognizing a Hemorrhagic Stroke
   ° Common signs and symptoms
   ° Importance of early recognition
   ° When to seek medical attention

°°Part IV: Emergency Response°°

4. Emergency Response: Acting Swiftly in a Crisis
   ° Calling emergency services
   ° Providing basic first aid
   ° Preparing the patient for transportation

°°Part V: Medical Interventions°°

5. Medical Interventions: Navigating Treatment Options
   ° Surgical procedures
   ° Clot removal techniques
   ° Other specialized treatments

° POTENTIAL OUTCOMES

°°PART VI: REHABILITATION AND LONG-TERM MANAGEMENT°°

6. ROAD TO RECOVERY: REHABILITATION AND LONG-TERM MANAGEMENT
° PHYSICAL THERAPY
° OCCUPATIONAL THERAPY
° SPEECH THERAPY
° CHALLENGES AND COPING STRATEGIES

°°PART VII: PREVENTION°°

7. PREVENTING FUTURE EPISODES: LIFESTYLE CHANGES AND RISK REDUCTION
° DIETARY RECOMMENDATIONS
° EXERCISE REGIMENS
° STRESS MANAGEMENT
° MEDICATION ADHERENCE

°°PART VIII: SUPPORT AND RESOURCES°°

8. SUPPORT SYSTEM: NAVIGATING LIFE AFTER HEMORRHAGIC STROKE

° BUILDING A SUPPORT NETWORK
° MANAGING POST-STROKE EMOTIONS
° MAINTAINING A POSITIVE OUTLOOK
° ADDITIONAL RESOURCES

CHAPTER 1

Understanding Hemorrhagic Stroke:

In the world of medical disorders, hemorrhagic stroke is a dangerous foe that can strike suddenly and have catastrophic effects. This first chapter provides readers with an essential overview of hemorrhagic stroke, including its definition, forms, and prevalence. It also sets the stage for a thorough investigation of the condition. An essential starting point is to have a basic awareness of hemorrhagic stroke before we set out on this quest to understand its intricacies.

What Constitutes a Hemorrhagic Stroke:

Intracerebral hemorrhage, another name for hemorrhagic stroke, is a serious neurological occurrence that is defined by bleeding inside the brain tissue. Hemorrhagic stroke is distinguished from its counterpart, ischemic stroke, by the rupture of a blood artery that allows blood to seep into the brain parenchyma. Ischemic stroke is caused by a blocked blood vessel that restricts blood flow to a particular area of the brain. Increased intracranial pressure brought on by this leakage raises the risk of brain injury, disruption of neuronal circuits, and a series of other events that may culminate in serious neurological impairments.

An Examination of Hemorrhagic Stroke Types:

There are two main kinds of hemorrhagic stroke: subarachnoid hemorrhage (SAH) and intracerebral hemorrhage (ICH). Intracerebral hemorrhage is the result of a blood clot that forms in the brain tissue after a blood vessel in the brain rupture, releasing blood. Conversely, subarachnoid hemorrhage, which is frequently brought on by the rupture of an aneurysm, a weak spot in a blood vessel, entails bleeding into the space between the brain and the thin tissues that cover it. Although blood leaking is a common feature for both types, its causes, methods, and clinical manifestations differ, which influences how they affect patients.

Hemorrhagic Stroke Prevalence:

The complex web of medical disorders shows hemorrhagic stroke as a powerful and worrisome strand. Even though ischemic stroke still accounts for about 80% of all stroke cases, hemorrhagic stroke is just as serious. Representing a significant proportion of stroke cases, it carries a heavy cost in terms of morbidity and mortality. Even with the progress in medical science and our comprehension of stroke prevention, hemorrhagic stroke still poses a challenge to researchers and medical professionals.

Building the Basis for Knowledge:
The foundation for a thorough understanding of hemorrhagic stroke is provided by this first chapter. The condition's diagnosis, kinds, and prevalence are all clearly laid out for readers, setting them up for further exploration of the complex aspects of hemorrhagic stroke treatment,

rehabilitation, prevention, and support in the following chapters. Equipped with this fundamental understanding, readers can approach the remaining portions of the book with a feeling of readiness and involvement, assured of their comprehension of the fundamental ideas related to hemorrhagic stroke.

As a result, "Understanding Hemorrhagic Stroke: An Overview" is more than just a chapter; it serves as an introduction to a complicated medical illness that can have a significant impact on both the affected person and their acquaintances. In this chapter, the definition, types, and prevalence of hemorrhagic stroke are clarified, enabling readers to go off on an educational, exploratory, and empowering journey. As we proceed, each new chapter will reveal more levels of understanding and direction, giving readers the resources they require to overcome the difficulties presented by hemorrhagic stroke and set out on a journey towards recuperation and wellbeing.

CHAPTER 2

Unraveling the Causes: What Triggers Hemorrhagic Stroke?

In this chapter, you could delve into the various risk factors and causes of hemorrhagic stroke. This might include factors like hypertension, aneurysms, blood thinners, and genetic predispositions.

An enormous medical disaster known as a hemorrhagic stroke happens when a blood vessel in the brain bursts and spills blood into the surrounding tissue. In contrast to ischemic strokes, which arise from a blockage in a blood vessel supplying the brain, hemorrhagic strokes induce a leakage of blood that can cause serious harm and even be fatal. It's essential to comprehend the causes and risk factors of hemorrhagic strokes in order to avoid, diagnose, and treat them effectively. This chapter explores the complex network of risk factors, such as blood thinners, aneurysms, hypertension, and genetic predispositions, that might cause this devastating catastrophe.

Overconfidence: The Quiet Killer

Elevated blood pressure, or hypertension, is one of the main causes of hemorrhagic strokes. Over time, the push of blood on blood artery walls can damage their integrity and increase the likelihood of a rupture. High blood pressure puts an excessive amount of strain on the fragile blood artery network in the brain, and when this strain becomes too great, it can induce catastrophic bleeding. Because of this, controlling hypertension is essential to avoiding hemorrhagic strokes. A balanced diet, frequent exercise, stress management, and, if required, antihypertensive drugs are examples of lifestyle changes that are essential for preserving good blood pressure levels and lowering the risk of stroke.

Aneurysms: Time Bombs That Tick Off

Often referred to as "silent time bombs," aneurysms are weak spots in the walls of blood vessels that have the potential to balloon out and explode, resulting in hemorrhagic strokes. These structural abnormalities may be inherited or may arise gradually as a result of a number of conditions, such as high blood pressure, smoking, and genetic susceptibility. Blood is released into the brain when an aneurysm bursts, causing an abrupt and serious stroke. Thanks to developments in medical imaging technology, aneurysms can now be seen before they burst, enabling early management. The risk of a hemorrhagic stroke can be reduced and aneurysm rupture can be avoided by surgical techniques like coiling or clipping.

Blood Thinners: Judging Benefit Against Risk

Anticoagulant drugs, often known as blood thinners, are frequently administered to stop blood clots and lower the risk of ischemic strokes. Although these drugs may be helpful for certain people, there is a possible drawback: a higher risk of bleeding, including hemorrhagic strokes. Healthcare personnel face a problem in maintaining a delicate balance between minimizing the formation of clots and avoiding excessive bleeding. In order to modify drug dosages and minimize potential dangers, patients using blood thinners require frequent supervision, routine blood testing, and close coordination with medical specialists. In order to reduce the risk of hemorrhagic stroke, people must be aware of the possible complications and carefully adhere to their healthcare provider's instructions.

Hereditary Propensities: Cracking the Code

The risk of hemorrhagic strokes in an individual is mostly determined by their genetic makeup. Some persons are more likely than others to rupture their blood vessels due to specific hereditary characteristics that affect the blood vessel's strength and integrity. Blood artery shape and function have been related to an elevated risk of hemorrhagic strokes by conditions such as hereditary hemorrhagic telangiectasia (HHT) and cerebral autosomal dominant arteriopathy with subcortical infarcts and leukoencephalopathy (CADASIL). Investigations into the genetic foundations of hemorrhagic stroke continue to reveal novel information and possible targets for treatment. People with a family history of stroke can benefit greatly from genetic testing and counseling, which can provide them with important information to help them make decisions about their healthcare and way of life.

Deep Down: Multifactorial Interactions

Although blood thinners, aneurysms, genetics, and hypertension are major risk factors for hemorrhagic strokes, it's crucial to understand that many risk factors often interact in a complex way to cause strokes. Lifestyle decisions that increase the risk of hemorrhagic stroke include smoking, binge drinking, and eating poorly. Furthermore, a number of illnesses, including blood diseases and vascular abnormalities, can potentially raise the risk of a vessel burst. A thorough evaluation of stroke risk takes into account various complex factors in order to develop individualized plans for management and prevention.

In summary, the causes of hemorrhagic stroke can be attributed to a complicated web of interrelated risk factors. Blood thinners, hypertension, aneurysms, and genetic predispositions are only a few pieces of the complex puzzle that contribute to this tragic tragedy. Our comprehension of these triggers grows with the advancement of medical knowledge and technology, enabling more focused interventions and better patient outcomes. The burden of hemorrhagic stroke on both individuals and society at large can be significantly decreased by addressing these underlying causes and putting preventive measures in place. More research and education will open the door to improved stroke prevention and treatment, as well as a better future for those who are at risk, as we continue to explore the intricacies of this illness.

CHAPTER 3

Signs and Symptoms: Recognizing a Hemorrhagic Stroke

This chapter would focus on educating readers about the signs and symptoms of hemorrhagic stroke. Discussing the importance of early recognition and seeking medical attention would be key.

A stroke is a significant disturbance that can drastically change a person's life course in a matter of minutes inside the complex web of human health. Hemorrhagic stroke is a dangerous enemy in this field that needs to be identified quickly in order to lessen its possible effects. This chapter illuminates the warning signs and symptoms that indicate a hemorrhagic stroke, acting as a beacon of awareness. We learn how crucial it is to seek emergency medical assistance as well as the significance of early recognition as we make our way through the confusing terrain of stroke awareness.

A Quiet Encroachr: Exposing the Signs:

A hemorrhagic stroke is infamous for happening suddenly and frequently without warning. In contrast to some medical disorders that may develop gradually, a hemorrhagic stroke can occur suddenly. In the rush to get treatment, it is critical to comprehend its symptoms. Although the location and volume of the bleeding can affect the symptoms, there are several common signs that should be taken seriously. Some neurological symptoms that may accompany these include a sudden, intense headache that is sometimes referred to as the "worst headache of my life," as well as dizziness, loss of coordination, altered consciousness levels, weakness or numbness on one side of the body, and trouble speaking or understanding speech.

The Critical Window: The Significance of Prompt Identification:

When it comes to hemorrhagic stroke, time is of the essence. The patient's prognosis and result can be significantly impacted by how quickly symptoms are identified and addressed. The "golden hour" refers to the crucial 60-minute window in which the application of suitable medical interventions can considerably reduce the degree of brain damage. This is a fundamental premise of stroke care. Early symptom detection thus turns into a ray of hope, a lifeline that may be able to change the course of a patient's recovery.

The Appeal for Intervention: Seeking Medical Care:

It is imperative that readers understand the importance of getting medical attention right now. The first thing that should be done when symptoms appear is to call emergency medical services as soon as possible. Prompt intervention has saved many lives, and this chapter highlights how important it is to not underestimate or ignore any stroke symptoms. It's an urgent call to action for those who are exhibiting symptoms as well as those in their immediate vicinity to take prompt, well-informed action.

Empowerment via Information:

The significance of this chapter is found in the empowerment it bestows as well as the awareness it raises. Equipped with the understanding of hemorrhagic stroke symptoms and indicators, readers take on a proactive role in promoting both their own health and the welfare of others. People can be more equipped to handle the difficulties presented by a stroke emergency if they are aware of the possible warning signs.

To sum up, "Signs and Symptoms: Recognizing a Hemorrhagic Stroke" proves to be a crucial section in the effort to raise awareness of stroke and provide early intervention. By delving into the various symptoms that define a hemorrhagic stroke, it emphasizes the significance of prompt diagnosis and the transformative power of immediate medical intervention. As readers take in this information, they join forces to combat the stealthy nature of hemorrhagic stroke, with the ability to recognize symptoms, take appropriate action, and possibly even save lives.

CHAPTER 4

Emergency Response: Acting Swiftly in a Crisis

Here, you could detail the immediate steps to take when someone is suspected of having a hemorrhagic stroke. This might involve calling emergency services, providing basic first aid, and preparing the patient for transportation.

An emergency requiring quick and coordinated care is a hemorrhagic stroke. When it comes to reducing the risk of brain damage and guaranteeing the patient's best possible prognosis, every second matters. In this chapter, we describe what to do immediately if someone appears to be suffering from a hemorrhagic stroke. We stress the need of acting quickly, contacting emergency services, administering basic first aid, and getting the patient ready to be transported to a medical institution.

Identifying the Symptoms and Taking Appropriate Action

Recognizing the signs and symptoms of a probable hemorrhagic stroke is the first step in treating it. A sudden, intense headache, weakness or numbness on one side of the body (arm, leg, or face), trouble speaking or understanding speech, disorientation, difficulty walking, loss of balance, and visual impairments are common signs of a stroke. Immediately acting upon noticing these symptoms, either yourself or someone else, is imperative.

Make an Emergency Service Call: Time Is Critical

Make an emergency service call as soon as you suspect a hemorrhagic stroke. The emergency number is 911 in several nations. Quick action from qualified medical personnel can have a major impact on how the stroke turns out. Notify the dispatcher that you believe the patient may be having a stroke and give them all the information they require, such as the patient's age, gender, symptoms, and any pertinent medical history. Keep your line open and do as they say.

Comfort and basic first aid should be given.

Several actions can be taken to offer the sufferer comfort and basic first aid while you wait for emergency personnel to arrive:

1. Remain composed: It's critical to maintain your composure and comfort the sufferer. Stress and anxiety may make things worse.

2. Lay the Patient Down: Assist the patient in taking a secure, comfortable lay on their side. If vomiting happens, this can lessen the chance of choking.

3. Don't Offer Food or Drink: Don't offer the patient any food or liquids. This is crucial to avoid choking and

guarantee that the medical team can properly evaluate the condition when they arrive.

4. Take Off Tight Clothes: To guarantee appropriate circulation, carefully relax any tight garments the patient may be wearing.

5. Observe Vital Signs: If the patient is cooperative and conscious, take their blood pressure using a cuff if you have one available. This information may prove to be beneficial to the medical staff.

Get Ready for Travel: Brain is Time

Emergency personnel will take charge of the situation when they get there, but you can help them by doing the following:

1. Give Information: Describe the patient's symptoms, medical background, and current medications to the medical team.

2. Assemble the necessities: Gather the patient's identification, insurance details, and a list of their current prescriptions, if at all possible. Hospital employees may find this material helpful.

3. Comfort and Reassurance: Keep giving the patient emotional support and assurance. It might be a scary process, but having you there can help.

4. Ensure Safe Transportation: First responders will choose the safest way to get patients to a hospital that can treat hemorrhagic strokes. Depending on the patient's location and the severity of the issue, either an ambulance or a helicopter may be needed.

Result: Taking Time-Sensitive Measures to Achieve Better Results

Time is brain when it comes to a hemorrhagic stroke. The patient's prospects of recovery and quality of life might be greatly impacted by prompt action taken in response to suspected symptoms. A well-coordinated and efficient emergency response can be facilitated by you identifying the symptoms, contacting emergency services, administering basic first aid, and getting the patient ready for evacuation. Stroke treatment is always evolving, but the importance of acting quickly never changes. You can make a significant difference in ensuring that someone suffering from a hemorrhagic stroke has the best possible outcome by being aware of and following these procedures. Recall that during a crisis, your prompt and well-informed answer can make all the difference.

CHAPTER 5

Medical Interventions: Navigating Treatment Options

This chapter could cover the medical interventions available for hemorrhagic stroke, including surgical procedures, clot removal techniques, and other specialized treatments. The aim would be to inform patients about their options and the potential outcomes.

Scientific progress in the field of medicine has made possible an impressive variety of methods to address the difficulties associated with hemorrhagic stroke. This chapter acts as a compass, helping patients and those close to them navigate the confusing world of available treatments. A wide range of medical therapies, including advanced clot removal techniques and surgical procedures, are available with great potential and promise. Readers that take on this investigative adventure come away with a thorough grasp of the various treatments that are available, their ramifications, and how they affect the course of recovery.

The Cutting Edge: Addressing the Wounds:

One essential component of the care of hemorrhagic stroke is surgery. Surgical treatments may be used to relieve pressure inside the skull, remove accumulated blood, and repair the damaged blood vessel, depending on the kind and degree of the bleeding. One such approach that may be used is a craniotomy, a surgical procedure that involves the temporary removal of a part of the skull in order to access the brain. This chapter offers readers a thorough examination of different surgical techniques as well as information on the advantages, disadvantages, and possible results of each.

The Development of Methods for Removing Clots:

There have been significant advancements in the field of clot removal methods for hemorrhagic stroke in recent times. Vascular operations, such coiling and stent implantation, have completely changed the field by providing less invasive substitutes for conventional open surgery. These methods entail inserting catheters and other instruments into blood vessels in order to get to the bleeding or clot-forming spot. Readers learn about the principles behind these strategies and their possible significance in minimizing damage and restoring blood flow through enlightening explanations and case examples.

Customized Strategies: Targeted Interventions:

Since every patient's experience with a hemorrhagic stroke is different, a customized treatment plan is necessary. In addition to endovascular and surgical procedures, specialty therapies might be used. This chapter explores potential therapies, including blood pressure-lowering drugs, brain-swelling medication, and possible preventative measures against rebleeding or more strokes. The collaborative efforts of healthcare teams to create treatment regimens that take into account each patient's needs and circumstances are made clear to readers.

Enhancing Knowledge-Based Decision-Making:

It can be difficult to sort through the plethora of hemorrhagic stroke therapy choices. This chapter's importance is in its ability to provide patients and their families with information empowerment. Through an understanding of the variety of therapies available, the benefits and risks that go along with them, and the possible results, readers will be in a better position to have educated discussions with their healthcare providers. With this empowerment, patients can actively participate in their treatment process and the decision-making process becomes a cooperative effort.

The chapter "Medical Interventions: Navigating Treatment Options" concludes by highlighting the critical steps involved in recovering from a hemorrhagic stroke. Through an exploration of advanced endovascular methods, surgical procedures, and specialty treatments, readers obtain a thorough grasp of the resources available to them. Equipped with information, patients take an active role in their own care, confidently and purposefully navigating the complex maze of available treatments.

CHAPTER 6

Road to Recovery: Rehabilitation and Long-Term Management

Discuss the rehabilitation process following a hemorrhagic stroke, focusing on physical, occupational, and speech therapies. Address the challenges patients might face during recovery and offer advice on coping strategies.

Hemorrhagic stroke recovery is a difficult road that calls for commitment, tolerance, and a thorough approach to rehabilitation. Following a stroke, a patient may experience changes in their body, mind, and emotions that affect their day-to-day activities. This chapter explores the process of recovery after a hemorrhagic stroke and emphasizes the value of speech, occupational, and physical therapy. We will also talk about the difficulties that patients could have while they recover and offer guidance on coping mechanisms to help them have a good recovery process.

Rebuilding Strength and Mobility with Physical Therapy

In order to assist stroke survivors regain their strength, mobility, and independence, physical therapy is essential. Patients frequently suffer from hemiparesis, also known as hemiplegia, which is weakness or paralysis on one side of the body following a hemorrhagic stroke. A professional physical therapist creates a customized exercise program to treat these issues. Patients improve their muscle strength, coordination, balance, and range of motion through focused exercises and procedures.

Activities that may be part of rehabilitation include:

- Gait training: Acquiring the ability to walk both with and without assistance.

- Exercises for strengthening: Resistance training to regain muscle. Enhancing stability and preventing falls is the goal of balance training.

- Functional mobility tasks: Getting comfortable with commonplace motions such as rising and falling from a chair or bed.

Adaptations and assistive devices: Acquiring the knowledge to utilize specialist equipment, like walkers or braces, when necessary.

Occupational Therapy: Gaining Back Your Daily Self-Sufficiency

The goal of occupational therapy is to assist stroke victims in regaining the capacity to carry out necessary daily activities (ADLs) and participate in fulfilling activities. This could involve activities like eating, cooking, grooming, and clothing. Occupational therapists work in tandem with patients to devise methods and plans that foster self-sufficiency and accommodate any cognitive or physical impairments.

Rehabilitation could include:

- Improving hand coordination and dexterity through fine motor skills training.

- Adaptive techniques: Acquiring knowledge about different approaches to challenges.

Improving problem-solving, memory, and attention are the main goals of cognitive training.

Assistive technology: Investigating instruments and apparatuses that promote self-sufficiency.

- Home modifications: Assessing the safety and accessibility of the living space.

Rediscovering Communication through Speech Therapy

Many survivors of hemorrhagic strokes find communication to be extremely difficult as a result of the impairments to their speech and language abilities. Working on speech production, language comprehension, and cognitive-communication abilities, speech therapists treat these problems.

Rehabilitation could entail:

- Articulation exercises: Improving pronunciation and clarity of speech.

The goals of language therapy are to increase vocabulary, expression, and comprehension.

- Swallowing therapy: Taking care of issues related to safe eating and drinking.

- Augmentative and alternative communication (AAC): Providing tools or methods of communication to people who have significant speech difficulties.

Difficulties and Coping Mechanisms

Hemorrhagic stroke recovery is not without difficulties. In addition to irritation, worry, and sadness, patients may endure overwhelming physical, emotional, and cognitive changes. It's critical that patients and the people who care for them recognize these emotions and seek out medical specialists, support groups, and mental health services for assistance.

Coping techniques consist of:

Setting Realistic Goals: Divide the process of healing into manageable steps, acknowledging and appreciating each new accomplishment.

- Creating a Support System: Encircle yourself with loved ones, close friends, and medical professionals who can provide support and encouragement.

Maintaining a Positive Mindset: Exercise self-compassion and concentrate on making progress rather than obsessing on failures.

Following Rehabilitation Plans: To maximize healing, follow recommended therapies and exercises; consistency is essential.

- Participating in Leisure Activities: Take up interests and pastimes that make you happy and stimulate your mind.

- Healthy Lifestyle Choices: Make attentive sleep a top priority, follow doctor's recommendations for frequent exercise, and maintain a balanced diet.

Final Thought: A Resilient Journey

After a hemorrhagic stroke, the path to recovery is difficult but eventually rewarding. Through speech, occupational, and physical therapy, survivors can enhance their quality of life and regain their independence. Patients and their caregivers can proceed with resiliency and resolve on this path by accepting the difficulties, getting the right help, and using coping mechanisms. Recall that each step you take toward healing is evidence of the human spirit's adaptability and development.

CHAPTER 7

**Preventing Future Episodes:
Lifestyle Changes and Risk
Reduction**

Beyond the treatment space is a proactive one where people can take charge of their health and set out on a preventative path. This chapter acts as a lighthouse of empowerment, directing readers through the maze of risk-reduction tactics and lifestyle changes that are essential to averting more hemorrhagic strokes. Modifications to diet and stress reduction are just two of the options available in preventive that have the power to change a person's health trajectory. Readers who follow this route of transformation acquire useful insights that enable them to take control of their own well-being.

Feeding Well-Being: The Significance of Diet:

One of the main pillars of prevention is diet. Individuals have the ability to influence their cardiovascular health, which is essential for preventing strokes, by making educated dietary choices. This chapter explores suggested diets, with a focus on including nutritious foods, lean meats, and a rainbow of colorful fruits and vegetables. It looks at how important it is to control sodium intake and emphasizes the advantages of heart-healthy fats. Readers learn that adopting a nutritious strategy that promotes good health instead of simply depriving oneself is the goal of dietary modifications.

Towards Vitality: Physical Activity and Exercise:

Engaging in physical exercise is a powerful remedy that can revitalize the body and protect against the risk factors that lead to hemorrhagic stroke. This chapter shows the transforming power of movement, from cardiovascular workouts that improve the heart to resistance training that supports muscle health. The prescribed exercise regimens are explained to the readers, who also learn that even modest, regular efforts can have a big impact on stroke prevention and general health.

Overcoming the Stress Paradigm: Stress Reduction Strategies:

Stress has become an unwanted companion in the hectic modern world, one that can have a negative effect on one's health. This chapter offers a number of techniques for overcoming the stress paradigm. Readers discover a toolset of stress management approaches, ranging from mindfulness and meditation to relaxation techniques and stimulating hobbies. Acknowledging the connection between mental and physical health, they adopt practices that promote peace of mind and fortitude, which in turn lead to a longer and healthier life.

The Journey of Medication Adherence:

Following recommended regimens is crucial for people who need to take drugs to treat underlying medical issues. This chapter explores the importance of medication adherence and highlights how it can help prevent hemorrhagic strokes from happening again. The tactics for efficiently managing drugs, resolving concerns, and keeping lines of communication open with healthcare providers are shared with readers. Through the process of managing their drug regimen, individuals protect themselves against possible hazards and enhance their overall health results.

Empowerment Through Action: "Preventing Future Episodes: Lifestyle Changes and Risk Reduction" functioned as a guide for empowerment and longevity, more than just a chapter. Readers go on a life-changing journey by accepting dietary changes, exercising, learning stress management techniques, and figuring out how to stick to their prescription regimen. Equipped with useful knowledge, they represent prevention personified, piecing together decisions that improve their quality of life while lowering their chance of suffering another hemorrhagic stroke in the future.

To sum up, this chapter serves as a beacon of proactive wellbeing where empowerment and prevention meet. Readers embrace the essence of preventative health through the examination of nutritional intricacies, exercise vigor, stress management finesse, and medication adherence dedication. This chapter acts as a spark, encouraging people to make decisions that have an impact much beyond the here and now, bringing in a future full of energy, resiliency, and the satisfaction of a life well lived.

CHAPTER 8

Support System: Navigating Life After Hemorrhagic Stroke

Conclude the book by discussing the emotional, social, and psychological aspects of life after a hemorrhagic stroke. Offer advice on building a support network, managing post-stroke emotions, and maintaining a positive outlook.

The process of recuperating after a hemorrhagic stroke goes beyond mere physical therapy. After an incident that drastically changes one's life, emotional, social, and psychological factors are vital in determining how that person lives. In this last chapter, we discuss how to create a strong support system, deal with feelings that arise after a stroke, and keep a positive view on your journey to a happy and meaningful life.

Embracing Feelings: Recognizing the Range

Following a hemorrhagic stroke, life can be incredibly emotional. Survivors experienced a wide range of emotions, from moments of victory and gratitude to frustration and regret for lost talents. It is imperative that these feelings be acknowledged and communicated instead of being repressed. Having open lines of communication with family members, caretakers, and mental health specialists establishes a secure environment for discussing the emotional effects of the stroke.

Creating a Network of Support: The Power of Connections

A robust support system is essential to a full recovery. Having supportive friends, family, and support groups around oneself can provide one a feeling of community and emotional support. In particular, caregivers are essential in providing company, advocacy, and practical help. Interacting with other survivors via virtual communities or neighborhood support groups can promote understanding and comradery.

Holiday Emotion Management: A Comprehensive Approach

Managing emotions after a stroke necessitates a comprehensive strategy that takes mental, emotional, and physical health into account. Among the strategies are:

1. Seeking Professional Help: Mental health specialists can provide treatment, counseling, and coping mechanisms that are customized to meet the needs of the individual.

2. Meditation and Mindfulness: Deep breathing exercises and meditation are two techniques that can support emotional resilience and stress management.

3. Using Creative Channels: Processing emotions can find a

therapeutic release through writing, music, art, or other creative endeavors.

4. Physical Activity: Engaging in regular exercise generates endorphins, which have been linked to better mental and emotional health.

5. Well-Balanced Diet: Both mental stability and physical health can benefit from eating a balanced diet.

Keeping an Upbeat Attitude: A New Chapter

Having an optimistic mindset is very helpful in adjusting to life after a hemorrhagic stroke. Even though there are obstacles in life, having an optimistic outlook can increase resilience and enhance quality of life. Techniques for preserving optimism consist of:

1. Gratitude Practice: Developing appreciation by concentrating on wins rather than losses might cause one's viewpoint to change.

2. Goal Setting: Establishing attainable and reasonable goals gives one direction and a feeling of purpose.

3. Participating in Social Activities: Keeping up social links and taking

part in enjoyable activities can improve spirits.

4. Ongoing Education: A sense of achievement and personal development can be fostered through pursuing new interests, pastimes, or abilities.

5. Physical-Mind Practices: Through the integration of the mind and body, practices such as yoga, tai chi, or qi gong, promote holistic well-being.

Final Thought: Accepting the Journey

Living after a hemorrhagic stroke is evidence of the flexibility and durability of the human soul. Through the promotion of social relationships, emotional well-being, and an optimistic mindset, stroke survivors can accept the process of healing and create a meaningful life after their stroke. Never forget that every accomplishment, no matter how tiny, is a victory to be honored. Remember that you are not alone as you start this new chapter; your network of support, your inner strength, and your steadfast resolve will lead you to a future full of opportunity, hope, and the promise of a life well lived.

www.ingramcontent.com/pod-product-compliance
Lightning Source LLC
Chambersburg PA
CBHW060756260726
48660CB00002B/641